1

THE ART
OF
DETOXIFICATION
AN INTRODUCTION TO MAINTAINING HEALTH IN A TOXIC ENVIRONMENT

Integrated Healthcare of
Montclair LLC Publications
295 Bloomfield Avenue
Commercial Suite 1
At Station Square
Montclair NJ 07042

ISBN
978-1-7339139-0-4

"To all those who believed me and in me when I told them what I saw - thank you, to the others who did not - thank you."

Table of Contents

Table of contents (continued)

Introduction

"Toxin" means poison for arrows. Although the term "detox" is too commonly known as "a procedure used on those addicted to drugs to assist them so that they are no longer dependent," a better definition is "the removal of toxins or poisons from within the body of any person." Specifically, these toxins operate on a cellular level often below our awareness.

If we are to "detox," then we are assisting the body in removing these toxins. It is an art form because, although we have some understanding of how it happens based on science, there are many clever, creative, lesser understood ways to assist the body to rid itself of these toxins.

In the year 1993 I came across some information while reading a book about cleansing the body. At that time I had no real knowledge of conditions on the planet nor that they could impact my health. I operated on a day-to-day basis completely unaware of the problems we all must confront or ignore. As a teenager I suffered from acne particularly on the upper back and the scars are actually still present to this day -albeit faded. I had no clue that what was happening with my body had a lot to do with what I was putting in it and the chemicals about.

I decided I would begin taking vitamins and see what would happen. Much of my life I had seen pockets of obviously dysfunctional people. I saw people who were addicted to drugs, who abused alcohol, who ate poorly, and in general who poorly cared for themselves. They failed to have vibrant skin, energy, and health. I then noticed that those who seemed to be "health nuts" who consumed healthy diets, took vitamins, exercised and focused spiritually and tried to eat clean, seemed to be happier, healthier, and they looked better. My whole life I'd been told, that when you're sick you go to the Doctor.

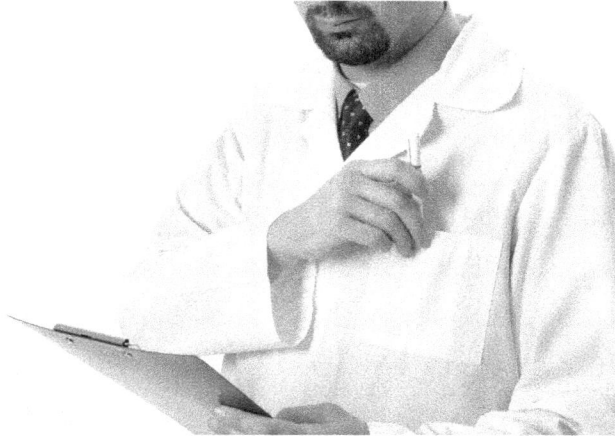

Illustration 1: Knowledge by practitioner varies.

I accepted this idea and also brought into the idea that "a real doctor" gave drugs as medicines. After all "what would be other reasons one would go?" So I took things into my own hands. I decided to go on an adventure which would change and redefine my life. This adventure and trek allowed me to assist in positively impacting thousands of people in ways that I don't even know about. I say this because "how would a fire inspector know if he prevented a fire if there wasn't one?" The following pages are very concise and a brief introduction to what has taken nearly a quarter of a century to learn by working with people, trial and error, and sadness and glory. It is meant to be done - practiced, not merely glazed over and set aside for later. First we will look into conditions with regard to the "war" against our health and look at strategies encompassing how we can deal effectively with these toxins and minimize the damage that's been done to us by ourselves, our foes, and our ancestors. It may come as a surprise that our inherited and very compromised ecological system is in danger and so are we. When you finish reading this work you'll be able to begin to understand steps you can take to start avoiding toxicity, as well as the ill feeling and illness that sometimes accompanies it.

You will know steps you can take to start to remove toxins trapped in the inner-workings of your body, You will understand what can be done to help your body stay cleansed and keep your defenses up, and you will know what to do to anticipate the toxic dangers about; finally, you will be able to understand one of the most important factors contributing to the toxicity of us all.

CHAPTER 1-
DON'T GET TOXIC

In the last 25 years there have been a number of wars that I've lived through. I was born during the Vietnam War and years later had to witness several of my friends fight in the Gulf War. It is interesting to note that the United States has been at war for 222 out of 239 years. Our military has been at peace for less than 20 years (www.inforwars.com). If there's one thing we can learn from war it is that a single war consists of many battles; and the longer a war goes on, the more fatigued its participants, and the greater the expense. That expense comes in many forms.

The more lives lost; the longer it takes to recover. A fundamental lesson from the study of war over the last 239 years is that since 1776 we might conclude that the best and most beneficial way to deal with war is to not get in one, to not start one, and to not participate in one. That is not to say that one should not defend himself or stand up for what is right. But when it comes to war an excellent strategy for winning is not to start one, and if it looks like one will start then negotiating so it doesn't should be the goal. After all, by doing this we could avoid the enormous death tolls, lengthy recovery times, and save leaving the legacy of countless future years of social and emotional turmoil. Based on the fact that these are the fruits of war I can only conclude that it's best not to get involved. I also have to acknowledge that there are times of war when it appears one had no choice and had to defend himself or others in an effort to serve a greater good.

The war on toxins is one you have been involved with your entire life. The fact is this war started in 1776 and has been being cryptically fought ever since that time. The environment has fought back and lost and is still losing. The casualties of this war are the ecosystem - "every creeping thing that crawls."

About 18 years ago the family and I decided we would vacation in nearby

Philadelphia. Tours of the city are really popular so we decided to go on one of the old "Duck boats." These boats were retired military "amphibious" vehicles that are able to operate both on land and sea. Transitioning "on the fly" is their specialty. In the midst of our tour, just as we begin to enter the bay going from land to sea, the guide pointed out that the bay we were entering had to be closed during the years of the founding of our country because it was so polluted. It was a sort of "ground zero" for the founding of the country and pollution (I thought to myself). I was very surprised when I heard this fact and thought - "this pollution is not only recent it is inherited and the accumulation of years."

Golden Years
Gold was once "smelted" or separated from undesirable contaminants with an unexpected ingredient. Smelting is the process of breaking down raw ore forms of

metals that had recently been mined into desirable constituents by ridding them of impurities. This is done using other elements and explained using chemistry's laws of attraction. Once the process is complete the waste products then must be discarded. Many of those waste products are toxins such as the metal mercury.

I also like museums and while going to visit an Egyptian museum exhibit could clearly see the Egyptians had a love for gold. They're one of the first well documented civilizations to use gold extensively to adorn themselves and their dead. The only way they were able to use the gold was after it was smelted. Their waste products are what we all have to deal with today - thousands of years later. Like others they used mercury. The Egyptian pyramids are thought to have been built 3,000 years before Christ. If that is correct the pollution of our planet started over 5,000 years ago and has been mounting ever since. Pollution is the price we pay for processing Earth's treasures irresponsibly.

Our toxic burden

So the first lesson we've learned is that there is a long history in this war on toxins. I only spoke of one or two of the many battles that have occurred and are still occurring. Our first rule to aid in winning future battles that we will encounter and ultimately winning the war is "not to get toxic."

So how does one "not get toxic" in a toxic world? Well the truth is, it's very easy to become toxic and volumes can be written about it. Since 1965 it has been. Ralph Golan MD, tells us that there are some 4,000,000 toxic chemicals that have been released and unleashed in our environment. We also now have electronically caused toxicity. This comes in the form of the physical components of electronic and magnetic devices. They produce a variety of energy that may be problematic. Some of the energies they give off are called "extremely low frequencies" (called ELF's). These frequencies may mimic the frequencies of cells that control the human body in some people. Especially in the brain. There is evidence that they cause subtle hormonal disturbances leading to sleep disruption and some cancers.

The truth is that at this point and time "not get toxic" really means not getting "too" toxic. It is important that we all get to know and understand what our toxic burden is! We all have a toxic burden, and it can be measured in several ways. Before I tell you the ways that this can be measured you must understand that in the war on toxins there is a "dark side" and a "light side." Everyone in Healthcare does not agree that environmentally caused illness is real, let alone caused by nearly invisible or camouflaged toxins. This is because different languages are being spoken by professionals and causing factions. Some people speak the language of "high levels of exposure" to toxins causing illness, and others speak the language of "low levels of exposure" to toxins creating illness. The latter is called "functional illness," and the earlier is an emergency room perspective – meaning if the exposure does not immediately make a person ill or does not kill them, then they are just fine. A person seeking assistance with illness caused by low level exposures would best be assisted by a Healthcare provider knowledgeable in the management of "functional health matters." Most of these methods of analysis require the assistance of a healthcare professional who understands that there is such a thing as environmentally caused illness – this is not all healthcare providers. Many conventional American doctors do not believe that such a thing exists as it was not part of their training.

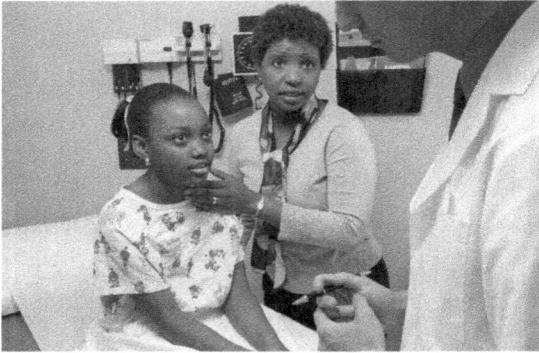

The United States, EPA's (Environmental Protection Agency) "gold standard" for the detection of toxic metals is hair analysis. Blood tests are sometimes used, and urine tests are also sometimes used to detect heavy metals as well. However, please recall that since 1965 four million chemicals have been unleashed and these go well beyond heavy metal toxins. In other words, there are many types and classifications of toxins. Based on this a number of tests are needed including a blood work study from a company called Genova Diagnostics called a "core toxin profile." This is a blood test that covers large numbers of commonly used chemicals that can negatively impact human health and function. While costly, it may be more expensive not to know that these are present in the body. How can you manage something that you do not even know is present?

These tests often times don't detect chronic low-level exposures which cause myriad health problems. And while chronic and low-level exposures are not likely to kill anyone quickly, most medical practitioners in the U.S. may not agree on the importance. This is because of their specialty and overwhelm in carrying out their basic duties. The work load does not afford them time to cleanse themselves of such ignorance. All one needs to do is look around. Toxins about have been

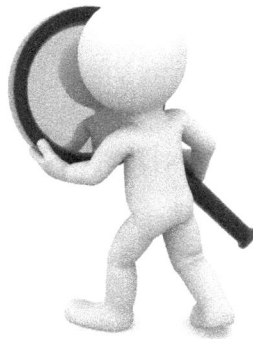

suspected for years of being the source of environmentally caused illness. They can be managed based on a practitioner taking a good health history and/or using various lab testing results. And in my 25 years of practice when addressed properly, health improves in many people. So to repeat the point, "do not get toxic" has to be modified a bit to "do not get too toxic." And one can achieve this goal by;

- by being vigilant;
- by shying away from excessive use of highly processed items;
- and by taking note of changes in health and how you feel and taking immediate action to correct this.

Just as one needs to avoid conflict and war, one also needs to avoid the toxins about. There are very basic and obvious times when one should be careful and this would be a good practice. However, there are also times when toxins are about and one hardly suspects a need to be aware or that these cryptic encounters can cause damage.

Here are some examples;
- pesticides on our foods and the food of animals we eat.
- the use of plastics in and on food .
- the use of air fresheners.
- the use of items that say the "fragrance."
- women's use of make-up.
- reusing restaurant containers.
- use of plastic that doesn't contain (BPA) Bisphenol A – A suspected toxin.

Below is a very basic checklist of what **to do** to not get too toxic;

- □ Eliminate or minimize the use of all plastic.

- ☐ Take note of how you feel around electronic devices. Some Applied Kinesiology doctors evaluate and support this imbalance.
- ☐ Filter water before drinking.
- ☐ Never get into a hot car.
- ☐ Avoid excessive consumption of restaurant food - it comes in plastic!
- ☐ Vote with your wallet and say why to restaurant owners.
- ☐ Vote for lawmakers who make the public health a priority and pass legislation that mandates companies' ideas and technological breakthroughs come with solutions for their toxicity

Chapter 2
REMOVE TOXINS QUICKLY

During times of war or a conflict of any type, it is probably best to bring the conflict to a halt as quickly as possible as the benefit is myriad. War casualties, deaths and turmoil wreak havoc. While war does build economies, it simultaneously destroys humanity.

Therefore, it makes sense to bring down such a juggernaut rapidly. Environmentally caused illness is substantial and the result of not addressing toxic exposures as quickly as possible. Ignorance here may be not only life changing, but perhaps life shortening, or in some cases prematurely life ending.

Such a war needs to have extremely short battles. The human body is set up to be a self-maintaining unit that requires fuel. The historical documentation shows that the human body is at least 3.5 million years old. It is designed to survive; it is a master computer and a master metabolizer - its design is unrivaled. The body has machinery intact that when not damaged has the sole purpose to cleanse and detoxify the body. The body is internally self-cleaning. Some of the machinery is listed as follows, but not in any particular order of importance;

1. skin,
2. liver,
3. kidneys,
4. Parotid gland,
5. and every cell in the body.

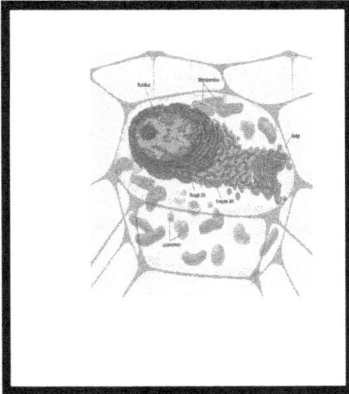

These organs and cells, in particular, contain microscopic machinery that is designed for the sole purpose of the elimination of waste products. Earlier, I pointed out that man has been around for at least 3.5 million years. The original waste products of the human body are those items created by the body but unused. These items left about, have the potential to cause "dis-ease," dysfunction and disease in the body. A few examples would be hormones that the body makes. The estrogen hormone is dominant in the female and the testosterone hormone in the male body.

After the body makes these hormones, there may be some excess remaining. The excess needs to be neutralized and this happens via a combination of encounters with the liver and other organs of elimination on a cellular level. The is "detoxification." The cells machinery would annihilate, deactivate, breakdown, eliminate or recycle these hormones. But left unchecked these excess hormones could overwhelm cellular machinery and cause a long list of "dysfunctions" such as acne, aggressive behavior, and untimely emotional behavior to name only a few.

So, for 3.5 million years plus or minus a few hundred, the body has been using its own god given internal mechanisms to maintain balance. It has been able to do so quickly and efficiently provided things were in working order. That is a pretty good track record considering most machines of the finest caliber such as cars get a one-to-four year or mileage contingency based warranty.

Unintended Use of Cellular machinery

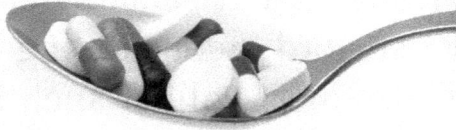

The first drug on record was made in 1900, earlier it was pointed out that four million chemicals and toxins have been released since 1965 - that's roughly 60 years from the time of this writing. So, in the last 100 years we've asked the body to use its innate organ systems that were developed over 3.5 million years ago for hormone management and deactivation, to remove chemical burdens forced upon it in the last 100 years? Fortunately, for most of us these cells and organs of elimination and detoxification have the potential to help and have stepped up to a degree and taken on the hefty responsibility of eliminating environmental chemicals from the body that if left unaddressed would harm it.

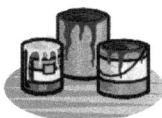

chemicals may cause illness.

When detox machinery does not work

Any person or professional who states that a person "could get all they need from the food" that they eat is not really cognizant of the current scene on our planet. And this person should not really be trusted in such matters. In order for the body's internal organs to efficiently eliminate toxins, the body must have the raw materials it needs.

The contemporary American diet, also referred to as the standard American diet (SAD), is devoid of vital nutrients. These foods have had their nutrients processed out. Organic or not, processing destroys nutrients. In cases where they have not been processed out, the food that is being eaten has been grown on soils which have been depleted of vital minerals and nutrients by poor farming practices and those plants had to be given a dose of pesticides to survive. Their innate ability to protect themselves is lost with poor soil nutrient content. That leaves one an additional burden of detoxifying their pesticide laden food after the intake.

A diet devoid of basic nutrition encourages slowed detoxification processes within the parts of the cell that would normally rid the body of its own toxins, let alone the additional pesticide burdens. Therefore the first major required step to ensure quick removal of toxins before too much damage is done is the regular and persistent pursuit of high-quality organic foods.

Ideally, these foods would be in their most basic form - unpackaged and not in plastic, fresh when possible, sometimes fermented, without preservatives. Examples would be apples, oranges, fresh meat (poultry, meat of any type, ethnic vegetarian protein sources, and some fish) In this rush-a-rush world people often ignorantly trade the prospect of health for the convenience of shortened time for meal preparation. If consumed the price of this is a blunted response to the burdens of our environment. This ultimately leads to decreased function of the body's basic maintenance processes, and "dis-ease," disease or disease like processes result. These may leave one feeling sick, dull, unhappy, and afflicted with mystery illnesses. To assist in removing toxins quickly, one needs to do the following;

- Avoid sugar, natural sugar, or sugar by any other name.
- Avoid prepepared packaged foods.
- Avoid fast and deep fried foods.
- Avoid processed white flour products.
- Consume foods in their natural state - instead of apple juice, eat an apple.
- Consume only freshly pressed natural vegetable juices.
- Avoid Caffeine.

There are also several groups of vitamins or herbal formulas designed to assist and these may be taken on a personal basis. They provide natural substances that aid the cleansing of the human body. This can be done and should be done on a maintenance basis as well. Doing so will assist removing toxins quickly.

Chapter 3
STAY CLEANSED

Now that you've seen evidence that the world is in poor shape and that each day we are all exposed to countless toxins you may understand why it follows that you should "stay cleansed." How does one stay cleansed you might think or wonder?

Recall from chapter 2 that the human body has a natural tendency and desire to work to stay in balance - it just needs help. This state of balance is constantly under surveillance and slight internal changes cause the machinery inside of our cells to go to work to re-balance the scene. It is all insensible to most of us. But is an automatic process.

A quick trip to the city, or through a puff of second hand smoke can easily start the body on a downward spiral if one continues on that path too long with inadequate support. However, if one were to maintain a natural unprocessed diet, lifestyle, and minimize the intake of sugar and manage toxic exposure by doing testing two times a year, then he or she would detect small problems before they become big problems. And the proper care of oneself alone would begin to thwart off toxic assaults. Please keep in mind that usually when one is exposed to toxins, they don't really feel toxic right away. Once the vital processes on a very minuscule cellular level are negatively influenced it is only then that we start to feel a bit off.

So if one waits for symptoms to act, it's already a bit late. Staying cleansed is a bit like being a professional in some type of career, sport or game. Professionals don't practice because something is wrong, they practice so that they can be the best they can be.

In addition to great a practice schedule professionals often look for "the edge." That something that will enable them to get better. The group of healthcare providers practicing using a method called applied kinesiology are an excellent "tool" that can be used to assist one in the detection of toxins or in getting that preventative "edge." This group are all doctors who are trained in a unique method of communicating with the human body to determine what it needs and what may be harming it. In combination with the list below this is an incredible healing opportunity and chance to make your care and prevention strategy individualized and more effective.

Since we're all playing this sport of detoxing and cleansing involuntarily in our lives and our quality of life is "on the line" we need to incorporate and maintain the following practices;

Daily

1. Expose ourselves to fresh air – 20 minutes daily.

2. Drink water - ½ our body weight in ounces daily.

3. Avoid the use of drugs and illicit substances – even if "natural."

4. Minimize our use of medicines when possible.

5. Take vitamins that we are certain we need (professional help may be needed).

6. Work to find the diet that is right for you. Some diets can cause a slowdown in our ability to detoxify if they're not correct.

7. Make sure toxic people are managed or eliminated from your life.

Periodically;

8. Go to your local Applied Kinesiology doctor for an evaluation of toxicity and your

body's ability to detoxify. (see references for practitioners).

9. Obtain an annual blood test that demonstrates your level of toxicity.

10. Obtain a hair analysis that demonstrates your heavy metal burdens 3- times annually.

11. Do not consume predatory fish unless you have your hair analysis done regularly and know your mercury burden.

By doing all of the above, you can increase the odds that your toxic burdens do not get out of control, and the levels are not too high. Then you can act quickly to reduce the levels so less harm will come to your body.

Chapter 4

ANTICIPATE TOXIC EXPOSURE

The true sign of a great warrior and those revered for their combat prowess in the past was that they had an ability to anticipate the enemies next move. Imagine for a moment if you knew what a foe or competitor's next action would be? You would go into action and you would cut off their next action because that would make you victorious. If you failed to predict or estimate their next action then you would receive what we call a surprise and a loss.

During war times soldiers would call this surprise an ambush. There's nothing worse than an ambush and the ensuing confusion and disorientation that comes about during and after one. Mentally and cognitively, there's nothing worse than an abrupt negative surprise.

The human body may not be much different. To ambush it with toxins means to overwhelm its cellular machinery. These overwhelmed basic processes sometimes become further impaired and ultimately sometimes lead to symptoms and illness days to weeks after exposure.

Once we apply the suggestions in chapter three any ambush will have much less impact because we anticipated. If one takes heed to the recommendations in this chapter, the consequences of toxic ambush can probably be lessened.

I'm sure that there are those who will read this work and think that anyone who followed this next chapter had some sort of obsession with being less toxic.

They are right! The goal and purpose of this chapter is to arm you so that you can better avoid the most common sources of toxins. If you can avoid these sources, you will have less to eliminate and less ill health.

But one does not have to be truly paranoid. There are some red flags that we all should take heed to. If done consistently we will be "grand masters" in the art of detoxification and win many battles by knowing our enemies.

What not to do

On a hot summer day a closed car is a potential menace, a toxic waste dump; it doesn't matter what model, or how much the vehicle cost was. The interior of that vehicle is loaded with toxic chemicals. One should anticipate a toxic exposure when they enter a car that has been closed especially on a hot summer day.

There's no such thing as organic fish. An otherwise fantastic source of protein and nutrition has been compromised by persistent consistent polluting of the oceans. Top concerns include mercury and PCB's or polychlorinated biphenyls. There are no organic oceans. If one is to consume fish, one must be tested at least annually to make sure that the toxic levels of PCBs and mercury are not reaching dangerous levels.

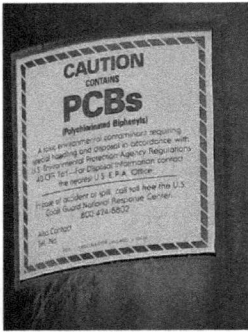

Photo 2: PCB Warning label

"Makeup" that women wear and "foundation" may be sources of toxic exposure. Each time women put these on their bodies they are increasing their exposure to xenoestrogens (foreign estrogens) in many products. It would be wise for women who wish to continue this practice to have their blood tested at least annually (for chemical forms of plastic, not just estrogen), regardless of what a manufacturer claims about the safety of a product. The laws of our land put the burden of proof that a product is toxic on consumers.

Have you ever wondered why after lawn companies treat a lawn they do not want pets or children on that lawn? What could they have sprayed on the lawn that would cause harm to children and pets? And what happens when it rains and it runs into the ground water? And then to the oceans? You can decrease the exposure of your children, your pets and yourself by not using lawn companies that have "patented secret formulas" that they are not required to disclose.

Keep in mind that regardless of the company or product that the weeds return every year! We are poisoning the plant for the moment, but the planet for lifetimes – one treatment after another. These practices and chemicals damage the human body and the planet. While not exhaustive, this is a list of common areas where people could anticipate toxic exposure.

- Consider the water you drink.

- Consider fish could be toxic to some degree farmed or wild.
- Does the company that sells product "x" say it is clean or environmentally sound?
- Does the product say "no BPA"?

Chapter 5
PREVENTION

"An ounce of prevention is worth a pound of cure." That is what Benjamin Franklin once said. And no place is it more true than in the art of managing the toxins about. We know that 50-65% of cancer is preventable, by diet, and addressing environmental burdens. In warfare when one wishes to strike a deadly blow to his foes with speed, the one area to attack is to cut off access to vital needs.

Vital needs include food, water, and shelter. Without these one becomes weak. What does it mean to our resilience and health when all of these are polluted?

Water

The human body is comprised of about 70% water. Water is needed for almost every process in the human body. Water when consumed lubricates areas, is an ultra solvent, and aids in the elimination of countless toxins via the kidney, skin, excretory glands (sweat glands), and feces via normal large intestine function,

If any routes of elimination are disrupted then so to some degree is optimal health. Water also is a major constituent of fluids that nourish and surround the brain. It carries vital cells essential to defense and immunity throughout the body. Water is the carrier of toxins and the major constituent of the final elimination of toxins from the body. When water is not present the human body withers as if a raisin.

Our bodies cannot thrive in the absence of water - it is the elixir of life and the foundation of this planet. While any water is better than none at all, there is no substitute for plain old water. Water is nature's cola, nature's elixir - a body fixer. It can resolve problems that other things cannot.

Let's get something straight; juice is not water, and water with taste is not water. Vitamins in water are not water, orange juice is not water, seltzer water is not water, only water is water. It is near neutral - balanced. It is defined by its narrow range chemically. It is not acid, and barely alkaline – a near neutral state.

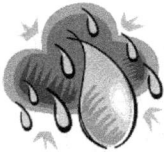

Illustration 3:

Once we add things to the water, it changes from its natural near neutral state into something else which has a different physiologic affect on the human body. If we are to truly detoxify, we need clean water. And by actual measurement our water is polluted even by government standards.

Government standards don't guarantee pure water they guarantee minimum levels of specific toxins by law. But only those toxins that it was legally mandated to test for.

What about the others? We know that over four million chemicals have been released into our environment since 1965 yet the standard for testing only involves at best one hundred chemicals. We also know that volumes of alarming information could be written about water that would seem surreal. It is an open secret however that our water suffers but most people do not fully understand to what degree. Those who want better health need to make good clean filtered water consumption a priority. There is much more to talk about on this subject but this is a good start.

Glyphosphate
pronounced Gly-fos-fate

If you recently saw a lawn care company spray a lawn or if you decided that you were unhappy with the golden flowers of the dandelions popping up haphazardly in your yard. Perhaps you then visited a local home improvement store and picked up "Roundup" or some other herbicide. With that decision you just joined the ranks of those herbicidal individuals who unknowingly caused and are causing contamination of the entire food chain with a chemical that has been implicated as a cause of cancer by The World Health Organization and declared the same - on and off (politically) by the EPA. These chemical residues are found in food – especially products that are not organic, and in the water supply and your body! Perhaps one of the reasons people without gluten intolerance do so well on "low carbohydrate" diets may be the result of the decrease in the consumption of glyphosphate residues not always the wheat itself. as it is sprayed on wheat, corn, and soy crops.

It is likely that every person in the United States at least, carries some level of glyphosphate in their body. This chemical is and has been the subject of intense battles and each time its maker Monsanto "legally" defends itself and somehow wins. Then the product use and apparent negative effects metastasize like the cancer it is believed to cause in susceptible people. The fact is the chemical destroys the very friendly bacteria that we humans depend on for our health and that definitely leads to illness and disease.

A urine test can be ordered so that you can know what your level is. There are several natural herbs and ingredients that have been purported to help the body purge this chemical. This was observed by measurement of lower glyphosphate urine levels after treatment. In my clinic we have created supportive cleanses to address this problem. We call it Glyphos-x.

Don't get toxic check list

- □ Drink filtered water.
- □ Take note of how you feel around electronic devices. Some Applied Kinesiology doctors evaluate and can support this imbalance.
- □ Eliminate or minimize the use of all plastic.
- □ Never get into a hot car.
- □ Avoid excessive consumption of restaurant food - it comes in plastic!
- □ Vote with your wallet and say why to restaurant owners.
- □ Vote for lawmakers who make the public health a priority and pass legislation that mandates ideas and technological breakthroughs come with solutions for the

toxicity they sometimes
cause.

Remove toxins quickly checklist

- ☐ Do a professional Detox Annually.
- ☐ Avoid sugar, natural sugar, or sugar by any other name.
- ☐ Avoid pre-prepared packaged foods.
- ☐ Avoid fast and deep fried foods.
- ☐ Avoid processed white flour products.
- ☐ Consume foods in their natural state -instead of apple juice, eat an apple.
- ☐ Consume only freshly pressed natural vegetable juices.
- ☐ Avoid Caffeine

Stay Cleansed checklist

- ☐ Expose ourselves to fresh air – 20 minutes daily.

- ☐ Drink water in the amount of ½ your body weight in ounces daily.

- ☐ Avoid the use of drugs and illicit substances – even if "natural."

- ☐ Minimize the use of medicines when possible.

- ☐ Take vitamins that you are certain you need (professional help may be needed).

- ☐ Work to find the diet that is right for you. Some diets can cause a slowdown in our ability to detoxify if they're not correct.

- □ Make sure toxic people are managed or eliminated from your life.

- □ Go to your local Applied Kinesiology doctor for an evaluation toxicity and your body's ability to detoxify.

- □ Obtain an annual blood test that demonstrates your level of toxicity.

- □ Obtain a hair analysis that demonstrates your heavy metal burdens 3- times annually.

- □ Do not consume predatory fish unless you have your hair analysis done regularly and know your mercury burden.

Anticipate Toxins checklist

- ☐ Consider having your water tested.

- ☐ Consider fish could be toxic to some degree farmed or wild.

- ☐ Does the company that sells product "x" say it is clean or environmentally sound?

- ☐ Does the product say "no BPA"?

<u>Summary</u>

In the next section you will be able to go get started on a basic detox. You should start right away. Detox for a 2-4 week period at least twice per year. Here are list of things you will need.

1. DTXmix – Full body cleanse From Harmonic Energetic s
2. Chlorolyph – Large bowel cleanser From Harmonic Energetics
3. Glyphos-x from Harmonic Energetics
4. Avoid sugar
5. Avoid caffeine
6. Consume at least 50 ounces of water daily.
7. Consume as much raw vegetable matter as possible.
8. Consume some raw fruit.
9. Decrease carbohydrate and eliminate grain consumption.

10. Stop meat consumption

Advisory: Always seek the assistance of a health care provider knowledgeable in detox and healthcare before starting any program.

References

1. The Art of War Sun Tzu
2. Synopsis of Applied Kinesiology 1998 David Walther ISBN-13: 978-0929721002
3. Understanding Pharmacology for Health Professionals, 5th Edition 2015, Susan M. Turley, RN
4. Guyton and Hall Textbook of Medical Physiology, 13th Edition
5. POPs vs. Fat: Persistent Organic Pollutant Toxicity Targets and Is Modulated by Adipose Tissue, Julia R Barnet Environ Health Perspect. 013 Feb;121(2):a61. doi: 10.1289/ehp.121-a61.
6. "Optimal Wellness, " Ralph Golan MD
7. EWG's Skin deep database https://www.ewg.org/skindeep/
8. The **Water** Quality **Standards** Regulation (40 CFR 131) EPA ground and drinking water standards.

Resources

1. Integrated Healthcare of Montclair, LLC - Wholistic,, functional medicine and environmentally caused illness. 973-744-1155 www.integraedhealthcare.us

2. The international college of Applied Kinesiology – Wholisitc functional medicine doctors, www.icakusa

3. Genova Diagnostics Labs
63 Zillicoa Street
Asheville, NC 28801
800-522-4762
Tests for Toxin Profiles

4. ZRT Labs
8605 SW Creekside Place,
Beaverton, OR 97008
866.600.1636
    Blood test for metals

5. Harmonic Energetics, LLC
   295 Bloomfield Avenue
       C5 Montclair NJ 07042
       973-233-0258
       For Supplements

6. ARL Labs Analytical Research
   Labs, Inc. • 2225 W. Alice Avenue -
   Phoenix, Arizona 85021 USA 602
   995 1580
   Hair analysis

Alphabetical Index

Glossary

A
amphibious – capable of operating on land and sea . Page 16.
Applied Kinesiology – a system of healthcare and functional medicine that uses responses from a persons body to assist in determining the correct therapy for for their body. It is practiced by licensed healthcare providers and usually uses multiple sources of information, including blood tests and history as well as the body responses to determine the correct path to take. Founded by Dr George Goodheart in the 1970's. Page 25, 49.
art – the expression or application of human creative skill and imagination. Cover.
B
BPA – stands for bisphenol A.

BPA is an industrial chemical that has been used to make certain plastics and resins since the 1960s. Page 24.

burden of proof – the laws of the land obligate consumers to prove an accusation against manufacturers. Page 46.

C

cell – The smallest unit of function in living organisms. It is alive and has in itself the ability to feed, expel, grow or die. Page 28.

cellular machinery – refers to the parts of a cell that operate to keep it surviving such as the center nucleus which directs the cells activities.

cleans(e) (ing) – (1)used interchangeably with detoxification; (2) a cleaning or emptying out of the intestines.

constituents – parts of a whole item. Page 17

core toxin profile – a blood test offered by Genova Diagnostics that looks for the presence of many common toxic chemicals. Page 21.

cryptic(ly) – in a secretive or hidden fashion. Page 15.

D

dark side, the – taken from the movie Star Wars, represents the evil side of things or evil forces, as opposed to the good side of things. Page 19.

detox machinery – refers to those parts of a cell that are designed to eliminate hormones and in the last

100 years have taken on the role of eliminating chemicals and toxins found in the environment. Page 32.

detox- Short for Detoxification. Page 8

detoxification – a chemical method used by cells of the body to eliminate chemicals, toxin, and hormones

doctor – a person awarded the highest degree in their respective field. In the truest sense means a teacher of that field.

duck boats – the DUKW (colloquially known as Duck) is a six-wheel-drive amphibious modification of the 2 1⁄2-ton trucks used by the U.S. military during World War II and the Korean War. Page 16.

E

ELF – Stands for Extremely Low Frequencies. These are the energy given off by radio and other devices. Since the 1970s they have been implicated in various health problems, including some cancers. Page 19.

emergency room perspective – the perspective that a patient only needs life saving care. This is the method of management in most medical practices. For example if one has shoulder pain and nothing is broken or torn, often no treatment or further investigation is offered except for drugs that cover the symptom and do nothing to correct it or determine the root cause. Page 19.

environmentally caused illness – illness that is a result of chemicals, poisons and toxins and such, present in the environment, food, air, and water.

EPA – "Environmental Protection Agency - The Environmental Protection Agency is an independent agency of the United States federal government for environmental protection. President Richard Nixon proposed the establishment of EPA on July 9, 1970, and it began operation on December 2, 1970, after Nixon signed an executive order." (Wikipedia). Page 20.

estrogen – the main female hormone responsible for female appearances and child bearing abilities SEE HORMONE .Page 29

F

fermented – a process where an organic item begins to be broken down or converted to a lesser form by the action of certain friendly bacteria. (SEE ORGANIC) Page 38.

formulation – (1)a method of preparing something or (2) the ingredients that make up a product. Page 45.

functional health matters – issues that deal with functional illness (SEE FUNCTIONAL ILLNESS). Page 20.

functional illness – sickness and illness that is atypical and does not follow typical medical diagnosis and often eludes traditional medical methods of detection. It responds well to drug-free healthcare methods and may make-up a large portion of illness in our society. Page 19.

G

glyphosphate – a popular herbicide that is linked to several health concerns, including cancer, and digestive problems. It is used on food and in any application to kill weeds. Created by Monsanto in the 1970s. It estimated to be a residue in the bodies' of most Americans. Page 55.

Gold Standard - what is believed to be the best and highest quality test result, or example of something that can be offered. Page 21.

good health history - health practitioners are expected to ask questions that clarify the nature of a patients concerns and illness. This is called a health history. Page 22.

government Standards – are standards for water testing set by lawmakers. These vary by state and government agency. Page 54.

ground water - "is the water found underground in the cracks and spaces in soil, sand and rock. It is stored in and moves slowly through geologic formations of soil, sand and rocks called aquifers. Groundwater supplies drinking water for 51% of the total U.S. population and 99% of the rural population" (Groundwater Foundation). Page 46.

ground zero – the source point or point from where something began. Page 16.

Gulf war - a conflict (Jan.–Feb. 1991) between Iraq and the United States and its allies to expel Iraq from Kuwait. Page 14.

H

hormone – chemical messengers produced by groups of cells (called organs) in organisms. SEE CELL IN GLOSSARY. Page 29.

I

Immunity – the body's defense system that consists of specialized cells called white blood cells, and defense weapons made by them called antibodies. Page 50.

innate – (1)in chiropractic , the spirit or that which animates the body;(2) inborn or from nature – natural. Page 32.

innate organ systems – are those ancient parts of the body such the cells which are under the control of a master energy source – the life force. Page 31.

J

Juggernaut – a powerful overwhelming negative force. Page 27.

L

light side, the – Taken from the movie Star Wars, represents the good side of things or good forces, as opposed to the bad or evil side of things. Page 19.

low level exposures – exposure to chemicals and toxins at an extremely low level – lower than what is thought to cause illness by the mainstream medicine and researchers. But is thought to cause illness by many alternative practitioners. Page 20.

M

maintenance processes – vital actions that occur in the human body on many levels with the goal of keeping it healthy and in balance. This is involuntary. Page 34.

make-up – a mixture of various chemicals and plasticizers designed to make a women look more attractive by smoothing the skin. The packaging and content of the makeup often contain questionable ingredients that may be harmful to the women and environment. Page 41.

Monsanto -"The Monsanto Company was an American agro-chemical and agricultural biotechnology corporation that existed from 1901 until 2018 when it was acquired by Bayer as part of its crop science division. It was headquartered in Creve Coeur, Missouri." (Bayer) Page 54.

myriad- many or several. Page 22.

N

natural – while this term means "comes from nature," it is used liberally in the USA as a marketing tool aimed at consumers who do not understand that many things are "natural" but unhealthy. This term has no legal meaning and can be placed almost anywhere. One could argue that plastic is "natural" as it came from fossil fuels that came from dinosaurs. Page 34.

natural sugar – SEE NATURAL AND SUGAR. Page 34.

nature's elixir – A remedy that knows no borders and has no limits. Page 50.

neutral – balanced, not negative or positive but in the middle. Page 50.

on the fly – idiom meaning while traveling of moving. Page 16.

organic- a term that simply means - contains the element carbon. Recently erroneously thought to mean healthy. However, things that contain carbon do not tend to leave a detrimental and long standing impact on the planet and pose a lower risk to life forms as they are composed of carbon in part as well. As such all can be recycled back to earth. Page 32.

P

parotid – a gland situated both sides of the head in front of both ears that is responsible for the production of saliva. Page 28.

PCB's (Polychlorinated Biphenyl's)- an oily chemical created by Monsanto and used in many applications from refrigeration to cooling transformers. New York City based Con Edison and others from the 1960's dumped these into the Hudson and other rivers and essentially polluted the world. They are implicated in cancer and other types of illness. Page 41.

physiologic – relating to function of the body. How it works. Page 50.

predatory fish – these are fish that fed off of other fish. They are fish eating fish. Page 40.

R

Ralph Golan MD - a general practitioner in Seattle since 1979, specializing in preventive, wellness, and longevity medicine. Page 18.

raw materials – nutrients, vitamins and minerals from food digestion that enter the cell one way and exit altered as a waste. Page 32.

Round-up – a weed killing product sold at popular home improvement centers and hardware stores that contains glyphosphate (see glyphosphate). Manufactured by Monsanto. Page 55.

routes of elimination – different ways the body can eliminate wastes. Examples are feces, urine, sweat, and vaginal discharge to name a few. Page 50.

rush-a-rush – informally speaking about people who are in a big hurry. Page 38.

S

SAD – Standard American Diet – this typically consists of potatoes, corn, string beans, processed meat, soda and sugar. Page 32.

smelt(ed)(ing) – to separate metals from each other to make one pure metal. Page 17.

Sugar – (1)a heavily processed

sweetener that has been altered from its original plant form and transformed into crystals or syrup and increases insulin responses. (2) Carbohydrate found in starchy and processed foods. Page 34.

T

testosterone – the main male hormone responsible for a man's deep voice, facial and body hair and muscle growth. Page 29.

toxic people – people who create trouble in our lives overtly or covertly. They may contribute to our unhappiness. That latter is very difficult to detect. But they must be managed. Page 39.

V

Vietnam War - a conflict, starting in 1954 and ending in 1975, between

South Vietnam (later aided by the U.S., South Korea, Australia, the Philippines, Thailand, and New Zealand) and the Vietcong and North Vietnam.

vigilant – alert and "on the look out" for danger or dangerous situations. Page 22.

W

Water – The formula for water is H_2O. That is two molecules of hydrogen and one of oxygen. This is water and if you add anything to it then the formula is changed and it is no longer water. It is the oldest drink on the planet. Page 47.

About the Author

Dr. Tyran G. Mincey is a clinician, holistic practitioner, lecturer, and educator from Montclair New Jersey providing applied kinesiology, chiropractic, herbal medicines, nutritional consultation, functional medicine based management, homeopathic and energy medicine, cleansing, detoxification, weight loss services, and Zerona cold laser therapy. A devoted husband and proud father of four children, Dr. Mincey is board certified, and earned his Diplomate in Applied Kinesiology, (a wholistic healthcare methodology) making him one of 48 teachers of this work in the world. And that includes 75,000 practicing chiropractors, 600,000 medical doctor's, 78,000 doctors of osteopathy, and 150,000 dentists.

He has performed over 200 lectures on the subject of detoxification and other topics since 2000 and is the founder of The Body Cleansing and Detoxification Center in Montclair New Jersey, LLC.

www.ingramcontent.com/pod-product-compliance
Lightning Source LLC
Chambersburg PA
CBHW031523270326
41930CB00006B/497